EAT THE COLORS

STOP THE KILLERS

God's principles for healthy living

Kwame Frimpong

Kwame Frimpong

EAT THE COLORS STOP THE KILLERS:
God's principles for healthy living

By Kwame Frimpong

For more information about this book, contact
Breakthrough In Christ Ministry
Website: www.breakthroughtoday.org
E-mail:info@breakthroughtoday.org

ISBN: 978-0-9849519-1-8
E-book: 978-0-9849519-2-5
Printed in the United States of America

Library of Congress Control Number: 2014923021

DEDICATION

I would like to dedicate this book to my Lord
and Saviour Jesus Christ. Thank you Father for
your grace, your love and mercy.
To God be the glory.

Kwame Frimpong

Contents

Eat The Colors

Kwame Frimpong

EAT THE COLORS: Stop The Killers

PART I:

Eat The Colors

INTRODUCTION:

STOP THE KILLERS

I wrote this book to help people who want to change their lives, be it losing weight, quitting a bad eating habit or simply adopting a healthier lifestyle. This book is for people who want to see a change in their health, but lack the motivation to do so. They feel stuck. Often people start out right with good eating habits, but then get easily discouraged, finding themselves in the valley of excuses. Then they give up.

Eat the Colors will help you breakthrough to victory over the barriers you face. My prayer is that the grace of God will help you overcome the odds and put you on the path to better health. I believe my personal testimony about how food changed my life will help you make better choices for your health.

Kwame Frimpong

In this book, I explain easy steps for weight loss using the W E I G H T principles motivational keys for changing your health. I pray that through this book you will be encouraged, inspired and fired up to take good care of your body, the Lord's Temple as Scripture tells us:

"Or do you not know that your body is the temple of the Holy Spirit who is in you, whom you have from God, and you are not your own? For you were bought at a price; therefore glorify God in your body and in your spirit, which are God's. (1 Corinthians 6:19-20)

CHAPTER 1

FOOD CHANGED MY LIFE

God spoke to me concerning my health (God delivered me from Idiopathic chronic thrombocytopenia and leukopenia)
"Plant more good seed to replace the space which the bad seed has taken."

In 2012, after I came back from Ghana, my blood pressure was 160/ 90. Now that may not seem too high to some people, but if your blood pressure has usually stayed around 120/80, you will be concerned. In addition to my blood pressure being noticeably elevated, my insomnia had also intensified. I had been averaging only around two hours of sleep daily for several weeks. In spite of the fact that all my medical reports proved negative, I became very concerned because my heart began to beat funny. I started losing my concentration and became very stressed out because I could not find any solution to my problem. I started praying to God to touch my heart and heal me from my insomnia.

A STRANGE DREAM

One day, as I was going through these troubles, I had a strange dream. In the dream, I was standing close to some bushes, when all of a sudden someone began to talk to me.

"Do you see these two trees?" He asked.

"Yes," I answered.

He continued, "Do you see any difference between the two?"

"No, they look so alike." I replied.

Then he said these words:

"Plant more good seed to replace the space that the bad seed has taken."

Then the dream ended.

When I woke up, I was puzzled as to the meaning of the dream. I immediately shared it with three pastors to see if any one of them had an idea of what it could mean. Without hesitation, all three seemed to arrive at the same interpretation. When I compared their interpretations, they all pointed to the work of God.

One of them explained to me that God wants me to keep on doing his work. Regardless of what I have been through, I should "keep on keeping on." The problem was that on the inside of me, I knew that the vision had nothing to do with ministry. After much prayer, I felt in my heart that God was talking to me about my health. He wanted me to eat more fruit and vegetables. Once I became convinced, I started researching more about natural food. I had been doing that due to how fruit and vegetables contributed to the overall healing of my mother's healing from stroke, but this time, I was in high gear. I took my juicing and smoothies to the next level!

Now three months later, my doctor referred me for more testing because he had discovered something strange in my blood. Well, on the day I headed out for my appointment, I ended up in the CANCER treatment center in Charlotte, North Carolina! When I entered the building, I did not have to be told that most of the people there were cancer patients. Now I started getting scared. So many questions flashed through my mind. Why am I here?

Eat The Colors

Did the doctor see something he failed to disclose to me?

What if they see something?

The questions kept coming, but I could not get answers for them. When it was my turn to see the doctor, he explained to me that they needed to do more testing. Something was very low in my system, and if it kept getting lower, it would be very bad news for me. Wow! I got very scared! They took samples of my blood, and told me that as soon as the results came in they would notify me.

Two weeks later I received a phone call. The doctor told me their suspicions were correct, and they would be unable to give me medication.

"What should I do?" I asked him.

Then he said this, **"Eat more fruit and vegetables."**

Kwame Frimpong

The doctor confirmed what God had already spoken to me in my dream. Six months later when I went for a follow-up appointment, the doctor said something very powerful to me.

"I do not know what you are doing, but do not stop!" the doctor said.

I believe the reason God told me to eat good seed is because eating junk is the main reason behind all the sicknesses the world is facing today.

Here is my first medical report:

Oncology Specialist

MD Chapman, Geoffrey S.

2711 Randolph Road, Suite 100

Charlotte, NC 28207

Dos: 03/26/12

Mr. Nyanor was seen at the C.W. Williams health Center in 11/11. At that time a CBC showed a platelet of 84000. The result was reported as "Increased Promyelocytes". Platelets are mildly reduced in number with many large platelets and a few small platelets aggregates.

Diagnoses: Thrombocytopenia, Leukopenia.

LABORATORY: Hemoglobin 15.2, White count 3100, normal differential, platelets 137000, HIV Negative; hepatitis C antibody negative

- By Geoffrey S. Chapman, MD

I started eating a lot of veggies and fruits, juicing and eating smoothies and below is the result of my blood work.

DOS: 08/26/13

Diagnoses: Chronic idiopathic thrombocytopenia and leukopenia

Kwame Frimpong

LABORATORY: Hemoglobin 15.7, hematocrit 46, White count 31000, ANC 1500, Platelets 102,000

ASSESSMENT: Chronic idiopathic thrombocytopenia and leukopenia STABLE.

- By Geoffrey S. Chapman, MD

On the following visit, my doctor asked me what I have been taken to stabilize my conditions. I told him I have just been exercising and checking my diet. He surprisingly replied "You are my only patient who is not on medication." Below is my latest medical report:

Oncology Specialist

MD Chapman, Geoffrey S.

2711 Randolph Road, Suite 100

DOS: 09/22/14

Eat The Colors

LABORATORY: His Hemogram is completely stable, Hemoglobin 15.8 MCV 89, White count 3100 with normal differential, platelets 103,000 - By Geoffrey S. Chapman, MD

Assessment: Idiopathic chronic thrombocytopenia and leukopenia stable since I first saw him 2 ½ years ago. There is no evidence of evolution to a more nefarious hematologic disorder.

Kwame Frimpong

EATING JUNK IS THE MAIN PROBLEM

(YOUR FOOD MAY BE KILLING YOU)

God created man in his own image to represent him on the planet. This was the purpose of God, so he gave Adam so much power to continue work in the world. We see this power manifesting through Adam as he gave names to all the animals. He was very creative, highly intellectual and prophetic. For this reason God gave Adam instructions to take care of his health. Here is his number one instruction:

And God said, "See, I have given you every herb that yields seed which is on the face of all the earth, and every tree whose fruit yields seed; to you it shall be for food. 30 Also, to every beast of the earth, to every bird of the air, and to everything that creeps on the earth, in which there is life, I have given every green herb for food"; and it was so. (Genesis 1:29-30)

As long as a person eats well, he or she will feel better, look great and is able to fulfill the purpose of God for his/her life. God also told Adam what to avoid so that he could maintain his health:

"but of the tree of the knowledge of good and evil you shall not eat, for in the day that you eat of it you shall surely die." (Genesis 2:17)

Eating from this tree was the downfall of man due to the disobedience of Adam and Eve. **And in our case, junk serves as the tree of death. The problem is we eat more of what we should eat less of.**

Eating from the forbidden tree was the downfall of humanity and, unfortunately, eating wrong food (junk) is eating the life in our body. Have you ever asked yourself why God told his people not to eat an animal with its blood? Here is what God said:

"And whatever man of the house of Israel, or of the strangers who dwell among you, who eats any blood, I will set My face against that person who eats blood, and will cut him off from among his people. For the life of the flesh is in the blood, and I have given it to you upon the altar to make atonement for your souls; for it is the blood that makes atonement for the soul." (Leviticus 17:10-11)

God told them why he did not permit them to eat animal with blood in it. Scripture says that it is because the life of the flesh is in the animal.

Now here is my point. Whatever you eat has life in it. **Either good life or bad life**. The junk we eat has bad life in it and it cuts our lives short. Here is something else I want you to see in the same scripture:

"for it is the life of all flesh. Its blood sustains its life. Therefore I said to the children of Israel, 'You shall not eat the blood of any flesh, for the life of all flesh is its blood. Whoever eats it shall be cut off." (Leviticus 17:14)

Notice the last phrase, "whoever eats it shall be cut off" in other words you shall die. I do not think that under the new covenant, God will kill people for not eating healthy. However, I believe people are cutting their own lives off by eating junk. It has bad life in it.

Also, God commanded them not to eat the fat of any animal.

"This shall be a perpetual statute throughout your generations in all your dwellings: you shall eat neither fat nor blood." (Leviticus 3:17).

When performing a sacrifice, the Levitical priests removed the fat, kidneys, and "caul above the liver" and burned them on the altar (Leviticus 9:10). It is our responsibility to look for healthy fats and avoid the bad ones.

GOOD FATS

MONOUNSATURATED FAT

- Olive oil
- Canola oil
- Sunflower oil
- Peanut oil
- Sesame oil
- Avocados
- Olives
- Nuts (almonds, peanuts, macadamia nuts, hazelnuts, pecans, cashews)
- Peanut butter

POLYUNSATURATED FAT

- Soybean oil
- Corn oil
- Safflower oil
- Walnuts
- Sunflower, sesame, and pumpkin   seeds
- Flaxseed
- Fatty fish (salmon, tuna, mackerel, herring, trout, sardines)
- Soymilk
- Tofu

BAD FATS

SATURATED FAT

- High-fat cuts of meat (beef, lamb, pork)
- Chicken with the skin
- Whole-fat dairy products (milk and cream)
- Butter

Kwame Frimpong

- Cheese
- Ice cream
- Palm and coconut oil
- Lard

TRANS FAT

- Commercially-baked pastries, cookies, doughnuts, muffins, cakes, pizza dough
- Packaged snack foods (crackers, microwave popcorn, chips)
- Stick margarine
- Vegetable shortening
- Fried foods (French fries, fried chicken, chicken nuggets, breaded fish)
- Candy bars

When it comes to dieting, I see three problems facing this generation.

1. **WE EAT MORE OF WHAT WE SHOULD EAT LESS OF**

Eating junk has resulted in a lot of diseases. Junk has taken control of man's life. People are so addicted to junk! People cannot overcome the addiction to junk because it is so tempting. Most people can't control the urge for junk food because they see it advertised everywhere! The packaging is very tempting and it lures us away, but we can overcome it and claim our health back!

Companies spend millions of dollars on television commercials. This is the same method the devil used when he deceived Eve. Satan made the tree appealing to her. Junk is very deceptive! The container looks great. It is often difficult to take your eyes off of it. We are what we eat, and we are poisoning our bodily systems with bad food. King Solomon put it this way:

"When you sit down to eat with a ruler, consider who and what are before you; For you will put a knife to your throat if you are a man given to desire. Be not desirous of his dainties, for it is deceitful food [offered with questionable motives]." (Proverbs 23:1-3)

2.   WE EAT LESS OF WHAT WE SHOULD EAT MORE OF

We need to eat more fruit and vegetables. You must include them in your daily diet. If you want to change your health, then you must make wise choices about your food. It is not enough to just stay away from junk. You need to eat healthy food. EAT THE COLORS! Eat fruits and veggies.

3. THE THIRD PROBLEM IS PROCESSED FOOD

Over processing and overheating destroys digestive enzymes found in fresh vegetables, whole grains, fruits and nuts and seeds. Overheating and re-heating vegetable oils makes them carcinogenic (having no potential to cause cancer) God has placed enzymes in foods to help with the digestive process.

In the words of Dr Colbert,

"The key is to practice balance and moderation, especially when eating meats. Also realize that this Scripture refers to foods God created. The foods that are causing disease and killing Americans are processed foods, fast foods, and foods high in sugar and toxic man-made fats and oils. Eating the right foods makes you physically healthy and wise.

Eat the wrong foods, and you open the door to degeneration, disease and an early death."

WE MUST RETURN TO THE COLORS

And God said, "See, I have given you every herb that yields seed which is on the face of all the earth, and every tree whose fruit yields seed; to you it shall be for food. 30 Also, to every beast of the earth, to every bird of the air, and to everything that creeps on the earth, in which there is life. I have given every green herb for food"; and it was so.(Genesis 1:30)

Eating fruits and vegetables was the first instruction given to man from God. Understand that God created Adam and Eve as his representatives on the earth to rule here. He needed to let them know how to keep fit, feel strong and stay healthy so they could do the job. So he gave him this first instruction

And out of the ground the Lord God made every tree grow that is pleasant to the sight and good for food. The tree of life was also in the midst of the garden and the tree of the knowledge of good and evil. (Genesis 2:9)

The tree of life was planted in the Garden of Eden, but we see it mentioned again in the (book of Revelation) end times.

In the middle of its street, and on either side of the river, was the tree of life, which bore twelve fruits, each tree yielding its fruit every month. The leaves of the tree were for the healing of the nations. (Revelation 22:2)

When you compare the two, you realize a big difference between the tree of life in the New Testament and the tree of life in the Old Testament.

The difference between the trees of life:

(a)   In the Old Testament, the tree of life was only one tree, but in the New Testament there are several trees of life on both sides of the river.

(b)   The tree of life in the Old Testament bears fruit, but the tree of life in the New Testament bears 12 kinds of fruit every month.

(c)   You do not have to wait for a particular season to eat from the tree of life in the New Testament because it bears fruit pretty much year round.

The question we need to ask ourselves is what is the purpose for one tree bearing 12 kinds of fruits every month? 12 kinds of fruit have at least 12 different kinds of colors. Why should the tree of life bear 12 kinds of fruits? I believe that if we were to take this tree literally, as in the Garden of Eden, then God wants to send a message and the message is clear, He wants the tree to produce so much fruit everyone would have access to it, because food can heal you as well as hurt you. It all depends on what food you are eating.

By putting a rainbow of color on your food plate, you will gain a healthy amount of essential vitamins and minerals. Here is what nutritional experts have to say about the importance of color in fruits and veggies:

"So what does color have to do with diet anyway? One word: phytochemicals. These substances occur naturally only in plants and may provide health benefits beyond those that essential nutrients provide. Color, such as what makes a blueberry so blue, can indicate some of these substances, which are thought to work synergistically with vitamins, minerals, and fiber (all present in fruits and vegetables) in whole foods to promote good health and lower disease risk." - Color Me Healthy

"Phytochemicals may act as antioxidants, protect and regenerate essential nutrients, and/or work to deactivate cancer-causing substances."

- Produce for Better Health Foundation

"Plant products are sources for phytochemicals of which there are thousands that have been identified - Kasik-Miller

"Eating a variety of foods helps ensure the intake of an assortment of nutrients and other healthful substances in food, such as phytochemicals, noting that color can be a helpful guide for consumers – Kathy Hoy, EdD, RD

"The anthocyanins that give these fruits their distinctive colors may help ward off heart disease by preventing clot formation. They may also help lower risk of cancer."

- Gloria Tsang, RD

Here are few Bible food and their benefits:

HEALTHY VEGETABLES OF THE BIBLE

Beans, peas, legumes

2 Samuel 17:28 (amplified version: brought beds, basins, earthen vessels, wheat, barley, meal, parched grain, beans, lentils, parched [pulse—seeds of peas and beans]

Nutrition facts: beans are one of the best sources of plant protein. All peas, beans and chickpeas are collectively known as legumes. Peas and green beans are both good sources of fiber.

Cucumbers, leeks, onions

Numbers 11:5: we remember the fish which we used to eat free in Egypt, the cucumbers and the melons and the leeks and the onions and the garlic...

Nutrition facts: cucumbers contain necessary minerals such as calcium, magnesium, iron, zinc, potassium, phosphorous, copper, manganese, fluoride, selenium and silica.

Cumin, dill, mint

Matthew23:23: woe to you, scribes and Pharisees, hypocrites! For you tithe mint and dill and cumin, and have neglected the weightier provisions of the law: justice and mercy and faithfulness; but these are the things you should have done without neglecting the others.

Nutrition facts: dill is a good source of dietary fiber and the minerals manganese, iron and magnesium. Cumin is rich in fatty acids, particularly the unsaturated and essential fatty acids (linoleic and linoleic acids). Mint is a glorious plant with intense aroma and flavor. It's in phytonutrients, vital vitamins and anti-oxidants.

Corn

Genesis 27:37 (amplified version): and Isaac answered Esau, behold, I have made [Jacob] your lord and master; I have given all his brethren to him for servants, and with corn and [new] wine have I sustained him. What then can I do for you, my son?

Nutrition facts: this ancient vegetable is packed with nutrients, providing fiber, which aids in digestion, plus folate, thiamin, phosphorus, vitamin c, and magnesium (about 10% of the daily value for each).

Garlic

Numbers 11:5: we remember the fish which we used to eat free in Egypt, the cucumbers and the melons and the leeks and the onions and the garlic

Nutrition facts: garlic is regarded as one of the most effective remedies to lower blood pressure, aid the digestive system, regulate heart rhythm, expel parasites, a remedy for whooping cough, and has been successfully used for a variety of skin disorders.

Olives and olive oil

Eat The Colors

Nehemiah 5:11: return this very day to them their fields, vineyards, olive groves, and houses, and also a hundredth of all the money, grain, new wine, and oil that you have exacted from them.

Nutrition facts: olives are high in flavor and monounsaturated fatty acids (the healthy fats). We know that low cholesterol is good. But none is better. And that is exactly what the humble olive has. Olive oil is a bible super food. The main type of fat found in all kinds of olive oil is monounsaturated fatty acids (mufas). Mufas are actually considered a healthy dietary fat.

Olive oil is rich in antioxidants, especially vitamin E, long thought to minimize cancer risk. Among plant oils, olive oil is the highest in monounsaturated fat, which does not oxidize in the body, and its low in polyunsaturated fat, the kind that does oxidize.

Pumpkins, squash and gourds

2 kings 4:39: then one went into the field to gather herbs and gathered from a wild vine his lap full of wild gourds, and returned and cut them up into the pot of pottage, for they were unknown to them.

Nutrition facts: the nutrient most shared by the squash varieties is beta-carotene. Our bodies use this to make vitamin a, which is essential for vision, bone growth and reproduction. The amount of beta-carotene varies with the color intensity of a squash's flesh. The orange varieties, such as pumpkin, are especially rich in the pigments lutein and zeaxanthin.

HEALTHY FRUITS OF THE BIBLE

Apples - (or *quince tree fruit)

Song of Solomon 2:5:"strengthen me with raisin cakes, refresh me with apples..."

Joel 1:12 - "the vine is dried up and the fig tree fails; the pomegranate tree, the palm tree also, and the apple or quince tree..."

Nutrition facts: fat free, cholesterol free, sodium free, good source of fiber, good source of vitamin c

Figs

1 Samuel 30:12 - and they gave him a piece of a cake of figs and two clusters of raisins. So when he had eaten, his strength came back to him; for he had eaten no bread nor drunk water for three days and three nights.

2 Kings 20:7 - and Isaiah said, bring a cake of figs. Let them lay it on the burning inflammation, that he may recover.

Nutrition facts: the fig fruits are important as both food and traditional medicine. They contain laxative substances, flavonoid, sugars, vitamins A and C, acids and enzymes.

Pomegranates (also one of the bible super foods)

Numbers 13:23: then they came to the valley of eshcol and from there cut down a branch with a single cluster of grapes; and they carried it on a pole between two men, with some of the pomegranates and the figs.

Nutrition facts: pomegranates are very low in saturated fat, cholesterol and sodium. This super fruit is a good source of dietary fiber and folate, and a very good source of vitamins C and K.

Dates

2 Samuel 6:19 - he also distributed to all the people — to the whole crowd of Israelites, both men and women — one loaf of bread, one date cake, and one raisin cake. Then all the people went home.

Nutrition facts: dates provide a wide range of essential nutrients, and are an excellent source of dietary potassium. The sugar content of ripe dates is about 80%; the remainder consists of protein, fiber, and trace elements including boron, cobalt, copper, fluorine, magnesium, manganese, selenium, and zinc.

Grapes (another bible super food)

Deuteronomy 23:24: when you enter your neighbor's vineyard, then you may eat grapes until you are fully satisfied, but you shall not put any in your basket.

Nutrition facts: (just a few – there are many) grapes are considered a super-fruit, having a rich source of micro-nutrient minerals like copper, iron and manganese. They are an also good source of vitamin-C vitamin A, vitamin K carotenes, and B-complex vitamins such as pyridoxine, riboflavin, and thiamin.

Melons a variety of melon was thought to have been grown in the Mediterranean region in biblical times.

Cantaloupe, honeydew, and watermelon

Eat The Colors

Numbers 11:5 - we remember the fish which we used to eat free in Egypt, the cucumbers and the melons and the leeks and the onions and the garlic.

Nutrition facts: melons are rich in antioxidant flavonoids such as beta-carotene, lutein, zeaxanthin and cryptoxanthin. These antioxidants have the ability to help protect cells and other structures in the body from oxygen-free radicals and hence; offer protection against colon, prostate, breast cancer. Melons are common in the Middle East watermelons grow luxuriantly in Palestine, even in dry and sandy soil. They are a delicious fruit in a hot climate, and were among the articles of food for which the Hebrews pined in the desert.

Kwame Frimpong

BIBLE'S LIST OF HEALTHY FOODS WITH PROTEIN

Lean meats of the bible

Lean is the key word regarding healthy meat. If you eat lean meat in moderation and also in proportion to an overall healthy diet, meats can help in keeping heart disease and type 2 diabetes risk factors down. Keep in mind, not all meats are created equal. The fattier red cuts provide excess saturated fats that increase your levels of LDL (bad) cholesterol. On the other hand, eating fattier fish provides polyunsaturated fats, which will benefit you by increasing the HDL (good) cholesterol, and supplying healthy omega-3 fatty acids.

Nuts, seeds, and legumes

Nuts: almonds, pistachio, walnut, pecan, and other nuts

Nuts are defined as dry, single-seeded fruits with high-oil content, enclosed in a tough outer layer. Some of their nutrients and fats vary higher and lower by comparison. Most nuts are high in fiber, protein and healthy fats.

Seeds: flax, sesame, sunflower, pumpkin, squash, and other seeds

Seeds are extremely nutrient-dense and they provide generous amounts of healthy fats, protein, vitamins, minerals and fiber. Seeds are certainly a nutritious biblical healthy food with protein.

Beans (legumes): soy, lentil, carob pod, black, pinto, and other varieties -

Kwame Frimpong

Beans are protein-packed, low in calories and high in nutritional value. They can improve health and ward off disease. Among all groups of food commonly eaten worldwide, no group has a more health-supportive mix of protein-plus-fiber than legumes.

CHAPTER 2:

NO MORE SALT

I have had a long history of migraine headaches. This started during my childhood and had persisted into adulthood. My pain would range from low level burning sensations on the top portion of the middle of my head to extremely excruciating pain. This is not fun! If you have never experienced migraines before, you might think people suffering from them are just making convenient excuses. This was not the case in my situation!

At the high peak of my migraines, the burning sensations would affect my left eye, ear and my left hand. Often I would just want to literally find somebody's belly to put my head in! Just like the woman who suffered from the issue of blood, I had been to several medical doctors. I was taking a lot of pain killers, but was without a cure.

I cannot remember the exact month of the year, but sometime during 2004, I became desperate with pain. Falling down prostrate on the floor, I began to really have a heart to heart talk with God about my migraine issue.

"When are you going to heal me of this chronic disease?" I petitioned God. I spent several hours praying to God for answers. After I was through praying, I sat in the presence of God just a while. From nowhere I heard or felt a knowing, or an understanding, or a voice.

You see, I could not explain whether it was a voice or a knowing. But it was like this: "no more salt." This experience was so strong, that when I told (Mary) my wife I would not eat table salt anymore, here was her response: "I do not believe that you could ever stop eating salt," she said. The reason she said that was because I had a habit of eating a lot of salt! And she was right! But what she did not know was that the impact of God's word had completely changed me instantly!

Three years passed and (Mary) my wife was shocked that I had completely gone without eating table salt and I never had another migraine headache. I did not know it was the sodium that was causing my migraine, and when I stopped eating salt, the migraines stopped.

LIVING WITH LIVER ABNORMALITY

Two years later, my yearly physicals showed an abnormality in my liver. My doctor referred me to UNC, Chapel Hill Hospital, to see a Herpetologist. That day, they drew blood samples for several tests. I was told to expect a call from Doctor Stephen Zacks in two weeks. One evening we had just finished eating dinner when the doctor called. He simply told me that, based on the blood tests, my liver was not functioning right. My liver function was abnormal, but there was no medication to help me. Then he said the situation was "not good." He decided to complete a liver biopsy and to monitor my condition.

My wife and I were very disturbed. Dr. Stephen Zacks arranged for the liver biopsy and he monitored my liver for 8 years. In 2010, he also referred me to a hospital in Concord, North Carolina for an evaluation. It was there they told me that I am suffering from Gilbert Syndrome. This is not dangerous, but I sometimes think I could have been killing my liver from all the pain killers I was taking due to my migraines. This is why I am grateful to

Eat The Colors

God for speaking to me concerning the cause of my headaches. Praise be to God!

CHAPTER 3:

ADDITIONAL TESTIMONIES

Drinking smoothies, walking four miles daily and juicing fruit and veggies cured me of 15 years of insomnia. I also did not have to suffer with (RLS) Restless Leg Syndrome anymore.

If you have ever suffered from insomnia (sleep disorder), you realize it is not a good feeling at all. Tossing up and down in bed and being unable to sleep causes a lot of health issues. You wake up feeling like your whole body is being beaten. You do not have the energy to do anything! Really, you do not feel sound at all. This has been my issue for many years.

You may ask: What is RLS? (Restless Leg Syndrome)

RLS is a disorder characterized by an unpleasant tickling or twitching sensation in the leg muscles when sitting or lying down. It is relieved only by moving the leg. The leg pain typically eases with motion of the legs, and it becomes more noticeable at rest. It worsens during the early evening or later at night. It may cause insomnia.

Usually you do not feel the tickling during the day. You experience it when you feel sleepy, and it makes sleeping very difficult. I did everything I knew to overcome this sickness. I tried putting soap close to my leg in bed. I tried lifting my leg up in the air. I tried many things! My doctor gave me all kinds of medicine. One particular medication even changed my mood for the worse. One day a friend of mine told me, "This is not the Kwame I know. What is wrong?" I told him I was taking medication, and he replied, "Then stop it!" That really made me stop and think, so I stopped taking the medication. Then I tried melatonin for sleep. It helped me a little, but I would wake up feeling like my whole body was on drugs.

I began to do an intense search for a solution. The first thing I found was that walking several miles a day could cure you of insomnia and that was it. I started walking four miles a day. Now I am completely free from insomnia and RLS.

BLOOD PRESSURE TESTIMONY

In the year 2012, when I returned from Ghana I knew I was under a lot of stress. My blood pressure was 150/90. It stayed there for about one month. I was very concerned because it was on the border line. I went to see my doctor for a checkup and they prescribed medication for me. But when I went to pick it up, there was a mistake with my name so I had to go back to my doctor. This time, they could not find my chart so I had to make another appointment all over again. It was there and then that I began to do research about natural ways to control blood pressure.

Now I am not under any circumstance telling you not to take medication, because you should. But I found out that drinking lemon and water every morning is good for your heart so I started doing this immediately. The results were amazing! The moment I started drinking lemon and water every morning, my blood pressure returned to normal. I have never stopped this practice.

Kwame Frimpong

KNOWING FOOD ALLERGIES HELPED
ME OVERCOME ITCHING

Another area of great concern is food allergies. You need to pay close attention to food allergies and realize how they might be affecting your health. My back used to itch all the time! That is until I met a good friend of mine at Bible School who advised me to pay close attention to what I had eaten prior to experiencing the itchiness. He told me to take a good look at things such as soaps, perfumes and food. I took his advice and one day, immediately after I had eaten a particular African food; (gari, beans and palm oil), I began experiencing the itch. I said, "Wow!" So I tried again another time, and realized this was the cause of my constant itches. I found out I was allergic to the combination of "gari" beans and palm oil.

Recently I had a week-long episode of RLS and immediately I knew what triggered it. I had been eating ginger, lightly salted peanuts and hot spices. Although ginger is a very healthy ingredient, I am highly allergic to it so I have to avoid it in my diet.

Kwame Frimpong

PART 11: BE MOTIVATED ABOUT YOUR HEALTH

CHAPTER 4:

I WAS MOTIVATED BY MY MOTHER'S ILLNESS

INSPIRED BY MY MOTHER
FRUIT, VEGGIES, WATER AND WALKING CHANGED HER HEALTH

Somewhere around 2003 my mother came to Virginia for a business trip. While she was here, she developed a pain in her lower back so she went to see a doctor. The doctor gave her medication for her back but when they examined her, her blood pressure was so high, she was strongly warned by the doctor to take her blood pressure medication. My mother had to go to New York the next day and she failed to take her blood pressure medication because it causes her to urinate so frequently.

The following morning, while she was still in bed, my mother experienced a sharp pain in her chest. She tried to get up, but could not do so. She felt like a part of her body was not responding. The following day she flew back to Amsterdam and without wasting any time she went to see her regular doctor. He ran several tests on her and when the results came in, she was told she had suffered several strokes which had affected her neck. This is what had caused her excruciating pain.

They started treatment, but her health was declining, so my stepfather brought her to the United States to consult with a specialist. When I saw my mother at the Washington Dulles International Airport in 2006, she had changed completely. She had lost a significant amount of weight and looked very sick which, of course, she was.

When I looked at her, I could not help but quickly escape to the nearest bathroom to weep. I quickly composed myself and then drove my parents all the way to Raleigh, North Carolina. After a few visits to the hospital and several sessions of physical therapy, Mother felt much better. Two months later she went back to Amsterdam. The situation gradually got worse again. The pain in her neck was so intense she could not straighten up. She could not sleep or eat anything.

She was still not well at all, but one day something awesome happened. A friend of my mother discussed my mother's problem with a member of the Seventh Day Adventist Church. Now, if you know anything about Seventh Day

Adventists, you will realize they are very particular about natural food research, and how it has shown that a natural diet leads to a long life. This lady came to my mum's house and brought with her a list of fruits and veggies. Here are some of the items on that list: Kale, broccoli, spinach, apples, bananas, carrots, celery, cauliflower, berries, ginger, peas, grapes, and many more.

My mother started juicing and making smoothies with the help of her husband right away. She did not quit taking her medication, she simply added natural food. Several weeks later she began to see changes in her overall health and now, over 10 years later she is doing fine. She has not stopped juicing, walking or drinking water. The change in her health inspired me greatly. Thank God for healing my mother through natural food.

MY SISTER INSPIRED ME

Diagnosed with breast cancer

I remember very well that it was in the year 2013. I had gone to Dallas, Texas for ministry. My sister called to tell me she was watching TV on the Ghana channel when she heard them talking about signs of breast cancer.

She told me she had made an appointment to see her doctor for a test because she had already observed something on her breast. She was told to come for the results in two weeks. During these two weeks she could not eat or sleep properly because she did not know what the outcome would be. We prayed several times on the phone and each time, I encouraged her to put her hope and trust in God.

Kwame Frimpong

When the report came in, it showed stage-2 breast cancer. It was a very emotional situation. We have never had cancer in our family before. We all cried and asked the question, "Where did this come from?" We prayed, and while we were waiting for the chemotherapy, we decided to look for a natural cure. We discovered sour sop leaves are one of the most powerful cures for cancer. My sister ate the sour sop food and drank the sour sop tea for several months before she underwent chemotherapy. My sister (Aggie) is still juicing, drinking smoothies, walking and taking care of herself. Her life is an inspiration to me. She is doing better today and we give God all the glory.

I encourage her to thank God for guiding her to watch that particular channel on that day in 2013. She could have turned off the

TV. Or she could have listened to another one of the 500 available channels on her television. But the question is, who made her watch TV on that particular day and who moved on her to turn to that channel? It was God. If God had not worked in her life, she could be dying of cancer unaware of her situation. Praise the Lord!

BE MOTIVATED BY YOUR FAMILY STORY

Your family history is crucial as far as your health is concerned. Every family has some kind of health issues going on. That is why doctors often have you answer long lists of questions about your family history. This is so they know how to provide you with the best medical care.

For example, my family has a history of headaches and high blood pressure. My mother had for years suffered from headaches and high blood pressure. My grandfather died of heart disease. My sister has also struggled with high blood pressure and headaches.

Now there are some people who succumb to whatever is going on in their family. They just accept it and live in default. They do not seem to do anything about it. They accept it, hoping that they will not be affected, but in reality it is just a matter of time before the hereditary illness shows up. Rather than just live hoping or wishing it away, I think that you can use your family history as a motivation to change your lifestyle. Someone and I mean you should break the curse.

Be encouraged to use your family history as motivation. Let it become the energy required to overcome inertia for you to change your health. When I realized high blood pressure was running rampant through my family, I made some drastic decisions which included quitting salt altogether. You know, by changing your eating lifestyle, you empower your immune system. This keeps your genes in charge of the diseases in your family from getting the upper hand.

CHAPTER 5:

TEAM UP WITH PEOPLE WHO ARE ON
THE PROGRAM

"Prove your servants, I beseech you, for ten days and let us be given a vegetable diet and water to drink. Then let our appearance and the appearance of the youths who eat of the king's [rich] dainties be observed and compared by you, and deal with us your servants according to what you see. So [the man] consented to them in this matter and proved them ten days. And at the end of ten days it was seen that they were looking better and had taken on more flesh than all the youths who ate of the king's rich dainties. So the steward took away their [rich] dainties and the wine they were to drink and gave them vegetables. (Daniel 1:1-16)

Daniel was not on his special diet alone, he had friends with him and they inspired and supported one another. Too often people begin their health journey very well, but they quit because they have no one to encourage them. If you try to get encouragement from people who do not have the same vision for their health as you do, they can discourage you. This is why teaming up or talking often with someone who is on the program with you is crucial.

A practical example is how Eve was deceived by the devil in the Garden of Eden. God gave Adam and Eve permission to eat from all the trees in the Garden, including the tree of life, with the exception of the tree of the knowledge of good and evil. But the tragedy was they never talked about the tree of life. When the devil spoke through the serpent, the conversation was never about the tree of life. It was not about eating healthy. Do you know why? It was the wrong conversation.

Why did the devil decide to talk about the tree of the knowledge of good and evil? Because he understands that what you talk about often changes what you will do. Satan therefore engaged Eve in a conversation with the aim to deceive her in order to eat the forbidden tree. The discussion was deadly! And when it ended, a seed had been planted in the mind of Eve. The result was, Eve ate the fruit.

This is the reason I talk a lot about doing things to improve your health. The more I talk about it, the more I am inspired to keep going. If you really want to eat broccoli, talk about it! If you want to start using brown sugar, talk about it and see what happens to your mindset.

My wife is very good at taking her vitamins. I get discouraged easily but she inspires me to take my vitamins. She, on the other hand, gets a lot of inspiration from me when it comes to eating healthy and exercising. Having a support group is crucial for your breakthrough in anything.

When my sister Agnes was diagnosed with breast cancer, she changed her lifestyle completely by eating healthy food and exercising. She always inspires and motivates me to take good care of myself. Daniel's friends, Shadrach, Meshack and Abednago, were all on the program: encouraging and inspiring one another.

King Solomon put it this way:

Kwame Frimpong

"Two are better than one, because they have a good reward for their labor. For if they fall, one will lift up his companion. But woe to him who is alone when he falls, For he has no one to help him up. Again, if two lie down together, they will keep warm; But how can one be warm alone. Though one may be overpowered by another, two can withstand him. And a threefold cord is not quickly broken" (Ecclesiastes 4:9-12)

Whenever I talk with my mother, we often talk about health matters like juicing, smoothies, taking a walk and drinking water. We also talk about new fruits and veggies we have recently discovered and their benefits. These are the things that keep me going. We end up encouraging each other.

CHAPTER 7:

BE MOTIVATED BY PURPOSE

WHAT ARE YOUR HEALTH GOALS?
DANIEL PURPOSED IN HIS HEART
CONCERNING HIS HEALTH.

"BUT DANIEL PURPOSED IN HIS HEART
THAT HE WOULD NOT DEFILE HIMSELF
WITH THE PORTION OF THE KING'S
DELICACIES, NOR WITH THE WINE
WHICH HE DRANK; THEREFORE HE
REQUESTED OF THE CHIEF OF THE
EUNUCHS THAT HE MIGHT NOT DEFILE
HIMSELF." (DANIEL 1:8)

Kwame Frimpong

The Psalmist prayed for wisdom about his health.

"So teach us to number our days, That we may gain a heart of wisdom" (Psalm 90:12)

In life, whether you like it or not, you are planning. If you fail to plan, you will plan to fail. You need to have an action plan for your health so you can take good care of your life. Let me ask you some questions.

How do you want to see your body 20 years from now?

If God blesses you with 110 years on the planet how do you want to be functioning at that age?

Do you picture yourself vibrant, energetic and strong at age 70?

Do you see yourself weak, tired and unable to walk at age 80?

Or do you simply leave it in the hands of God? Remember that God created nature but we are responsible for the environment.

The time to plan for your health is now. You may argue that it's hard to have time for your health with your busy schedule, but the amazing thing about Daniel was he was not completely in charge of his life, yet he had a purpose for his health. He was a slave, but he did not allow that to take his God-given choice away. He was disciplined enough to have a goal for his health.

I am sure it was not easy for Daniel to have this purpose in Babylon. It required discipline and determination. Some of you live by yourself and no one tells you what do to, and yet you fail to plan. Daniel did not have complete freedom. Someone told him what to eat, when to eat and how much he could eat. Yet he had a plan.

Purpose is so powerful! Daniel's purpose helped him overcome all the odds. You can overcome the odds too by having a purpose for your health, by using good planning and by asking God for His grace. You can do it too! No amount of junk food tempting you left and right can stop you from the purpose of God for your life.

Your body is a temple! Take care of it!

CHAPTER 8:

BE MOTIVATED BY THE IMPROVEMENTS IN YOUR HEALTH

Test us for 10 days.

"And at the end of ten days their features appeared better and fatter in flesh than all the young men who ate the portion of the king's delicacies" (Daniel 1:15)

At the end of ten days, the supervisor of Daniel and his friends saw a big difference in them far better than all the others and as a result he did not bother them about eating the king's food any more. King Nebuchadnezzar himself testified of this:

Kwame Frimpong

"Then the king interviewed[b] them, and among them all none was found like Daniel, Hananiah, Mishael, and Azariah; therefore they served before the king. And in all matters of wisdom and understanding about which the king examined them, he found them ten times better than all the magicians and astrologers who were in all his realm" (Daniel 1:19-20)

People ask me all the time:

"Are you still drinking your lemon water in the morning?"

"Are you still doing your 4 mile walk daily?"

And my answer has always been, "Yes, by the grace of God I am." Do you wonder what keeps me going? It is simply the improvements I see in my health and the grace of God.

If you have ever struggled to sleep and have been unable to do so, once you find a solution you won't quit. If you have had constant migraine headaches for years, and God shows you the cause and the cure, you won't give it up!

The lifestyle changes I have made in my life including drinking 48 ounce of water with honey and lemon daily, walking four miles daily, making smoothies and juicing, and giving up eating salt have made an enormous difference in my health.

I sleep better, I do not suffer with Restless Leg Syndrome anymore, the migraine has stopped and I feel great.

I think more clearly because of the grace of God which enables me to keep on with a healthy lifestyle. The Scripture says that at the end of ten days when Daniel and his friends were tested, they were ten times better than all those eating from the king's table. Why would you stop the program when you are ten times better off than those around you? Why would you stop when you feel better? Why would you stop when you look better? Why would you stop when you think better? If it is working, then keep on going!

CHAPTER 9:

MOTIVATED BY NATURAL THINGS GOD USES FOR SPIRITUAL TRUTH

The Bible is full of analogies that are very revealing when it comes to health. People who are very serious about their health notice these analogies. God is mindful of good health. He would not use something harmful to explain a spiritual truth. Therefore, if he uses natural things to explain spiritual truth, then it means those things have parallel truths too.

Consider the following analogies:

God will not use something harmful to teach you a spiritual truth as far as your health is concerned. For example, I don't think God will use something bad in order to teach us something good.

Kwame Frimpong

1)   Man's life is compared to the life of a tree:

"They shall not build and another inhabit; they shall not plant and another eat [the fruit]. For as the days of a tree, so shall be the days of My people, and My chosen and elect shall long make use of and enjoy the work of their hands." (Isaiah 65:22)

2)   God uses "walking" as a journey to perfection and wholeness:

"When Abram was ninety-nine years old, the Lord appeared to him and said, 'I am God Almighty; walk before me faithfully and be blameless." (Gen 17:1)

"And Enoch walked with God; and he was not, for God took him" (Gen 5:24)

God uses a "land flowing with milk and honey" 17 times to describe a land of plenty and good things. Unfortunately, our society has changed it to a land of soda, pop and candy.

"So I have come down to deliver them out of the hand of the Egyptians, and to bring them up from that land to a good and large land, to a land flowing with milk and honey, to the place of the Canaanites and the Hittites and the Amorites and the Perizzites and the Hivites and the Jebusites." (Exodus 3:8)

3)   Rivers of living waters

"He that believeth on me, as the scripture hath said, out of his belly shall flow rivers of living water." (John 7:38)

 Pomegranate in the temple

a)   "A golden bell and a pomegranate, a golden bell and a pomegranate, upon the hem of the robe round about." (Exodus 28:34)

b)   "A bell and a pomegranate, a bell and a pomegranate, all around the hem of the robe to minister in, as the Lord had commanded Moses." (Exodus 39:26)

Here is a list of the benefits of pomegranate:

• Most powerful anti-oxidant of all fruits

• Potent anti-cancer and immune supporting effects

• Inhibits abnormal platelet aggregation that could cause heart attacks, strokes and embolic disease

• Lowers cholesterol and other cardiac risk factors

• Lowers blood pressure

• Shown to promote reversal of atherosclerotic plaque in human studies

•   May have benefits to relieve or protect against depression and osteoporosis

4)   The olive leaf came out first after the flood of Noah

a)   "Then the dove came to him in the evening, and behold, a freshly plucked olive leaf was in her mouth; and Noah knew that the waters had receded from the

earth" (Genesis 8:11)

"Extra virgin olive oil is highly beneficial for our body. It works to promote heart health and also reduces the risk of developing various kinds of cancer."

– Dr Colbert

5)   Myrtle tree

Kwame Frimpong

a) "Instead of the thorn shall come up the cypress tree, And instead of the brier shall come up the myrtle tree; And it shall be to the Lord for a name, For an everlasting sign that shall not be cut off." (Isaiah 55:13)

This property of myrtle oil reduces the presence and further deposition of phlegm. It also clears congestion of the nasal tracts, bronchi and lungs resulting from colds and provides good relief from coughing(organic facts)

6)   Fruit as a blessing

a)   "This is what the Lord says:"As when juice is still found in a cluster of grapes and people say, 'Don't destroy it, there is still a blessing in it, 'so will I do on behalf of my servants; I will not destroy them all." (Isaiah 65:8 9) (NIV)

7)   Almond tree

a)   "The word of the Lord came to me: "What do you see, Jeremiah?" I see the branch of an almond tree," I replied. The Lord said to me, "You have seen correctly, for I am watching[a] to see that my word is fulfilled."

(Jeremiah 1:1-12)

8)   Mulberry tree

a) "Therefore David inquired of the Lord, and He said, "You shall not go up; circle around behind them, and come upon them in front of the mulberry trees. 24 And it shall be, when you hear the sound of marching in the tops of the mulberry trees, then you shall advance quickly. For then the Lord will go out before you to strike the camp of the Philistines." (2 Sam 5:23-25)

Ezekiel, the prophet had a vision which has spiritual meaning. However, we can take lessons from the natural things God used in visions and learn from them. The Bible mentions several natural things that are good for you if you practice them.

1.   Walking through the water or swimming (Ezekiel 47:1-5). There are several times that God uses walking for spiritual truths:

a.   Walk through the land-(Genesis 13:17)

b.   Walk before me and be perfect (Genesis 17:1)

c.   That you might walk worthy of the Lord unto all pleasing being fruitful in every god work and increasing in the knowledge of walk. (Colossians 1:10)

Key word: Walking. Walking is important exercise. Start walking and see a change in your health. I try to walk four miles daily.

2.   Water: Ezekiel 47:1-5. Water for healing: Ezekiel 47:9

a.   "On the last day, that great day of the feast, Jesus stood and cried out, saying, "If anyone thirsts, let him come to Me and drink. 38 He who believes in Me, as the Scripture has said, out of his heart will flow rivers of living water." (John 7:37)

b.   "Now a river went out of Eden to water the garden, and from there it parted and became four riverheads. 11 The name of the first is Pishon; it is the one which skirts the whole land of Havilah, where there is gold. 12

And the gold of that land is good. Bdellium and the onyx stone are there. 13 The name of the second river is Gihon; it is the one which goes around the whole land of Cush. 14 The name of the third river is Hiddekel;[b] it is the one which goes toward the east of Assyria. The fourth river is the Euphrates." (Genesis 2:10-14)

c.   "And he showed me a pure[a] river of water of life, clear as crystal, proceeding from the throne of God and of the Lamb" (Revelation 22:1)

Key word: Water. Water is good for you, 75% of both your brain and your entire body is water. You are supposed to drink water according to half of your body weight.

3.   Fruit (Ezekiel 47:12)

a.   "In the middle of its street, and on either side of the river, was the tree of life, which bore twelve fruits, each tree yielding its fruit every month. The leaves of the tree were for the healing of the nations." (Revelation 22:2)

Key word: Fruit. Fruit is good for you.

4.   Leaf (Ezekiel 47:12)

a.   And God said, "See, I have given you every herb that yields seed which is on the face of all the earth, and every tree whose fruit yields seed; to you it shall be for food. (Genesis 1:29)

5.   Fish in the sea.

a. "And it shall be that every living thing that moves, wherever the rivers go, will live. There will be a very great multitude of fish, because these waters go there; for they will be healed, and everything will live wherever the river goes" (Ezekiel 47:9)

PART III

CHAPTER 10: MOTIVATED BY THE NEW TESTAMENT CHALLENGE

"For no man ever yet hated his own flesh; but nourisheth and cherisheth it, even as the Lord the church" (Ephesians 5:29)

God has given us two responsibilities for our health: we are to nourish our bodies and cherish them. What I have often seen in the body of Christ is this: A lot of times people want God to do for them what he has already said in his word they are responsible to do. Here is a good example: Sometimes people just want to pray and have faith that God will take care of their health. And He does! He does by showing us what our responsibility is. He has also given us a clear responsibility to take care of our health.

The first responsibility is to nourish your body. Let's find the meaning of the word "nourishment." It means to sustain with food or nutriment. To supply with what is necessary for life, health, and growth. Cherish means this: To keep alive. To hold or treat as dear. To care for tenderly. To nurture. Now that we know the meaning two words, the question becomes, do we really care for our bodies?

Here is what I call the "New Testament Challenge." The Scriptures says, "No man hates his body." Let me ask you a few questions:

Do you really love your body?

How do you even know if you love your body?

Do you also know that God wants you to love your body?

How do you not hate your body?

Well from this text we can say there are at least two ways you can show that you love your body and that you take good care of it. Here are the two ways: nourishment and cherishment. The question is: how are you nourishing your body?

God has given you the responsibility to take care of your body. Sometimes out of laziness, believers have the tendency to leave out the part they need to play as far as health is concerned. They junk their system because of their belief in the blood of Jesus to take care of them.

Well, we know the blood of Jesus takes care of us. There is power in the blood to heal

(Isaiah 53) but it does not mean we should just eat junk!

NEW TESTAMENT FOOD VS.: OLD TESTAMENT FOOD: FINDING CLARITY

The Israelites were given a set of Dietary Laws at Mount Sinai. These were recorded by Moses. They are found in Leviticus chapter 11 and Deuteronomy chapter 14. In the New Testament, there are no prescribed foods:

Food controversy

(1)   Peter's dream

"And saw heaven opened and an object like a great sheet bound at the four corners, descending to him and let down to the earth. In it were all kinds of four-footed animals of the earth, wild beasts, creeping things, and birds of the air. 13 And a voice came to him, "Rise, Peter; kill and eat." But Peter said, "Not so, Lord! For I have never eaten anything common or unclean" (Acts 10:11-14)

Does the vision of Peter make all meat clean? Why was he still trying to figure out what the dream meant? If God wanted him to understand that he now considers all meat clean, it had nothing to do with Jewish diet. It had to do with the gospel to the Gentiles.

If God abolished the clean and unclean birds, why would he judge people based on that in the last days?

"For behold, the Lord will come with fire and with His chariots, like a whirlwind, to render His anger with fury, And His rebuke with flames of fire. For by fire and by His sword The Lord will judge all flesh; And the slain of the Lord shall be many. Those who sanctify themselves and purify themselves, To go to the gardens After an idol in the midst, Eating swine's flesh and the abomination and the mouse, Shall be consumed together," says the Lord."(Isaiah: 66:15-17)

Questions:

Does God still recognize clean and unclean foods?

If yes, why did He tell Peter that all birds are clean?

Are all foods clean?

"Men who forbid marriage and advocate abstaining from foods which God has created to be gratefully shared in by those who believe and know the truth. For everything created by God is good, and nothing is to be rejected if it is received with gratitude; 5 for it is sanctified by means of the word of God and prayer."Ist Tim 4:3-5((NASB)

Kwame Frimpong

Many people use this scripture to consider all food clean, so let us discuss few points here.

Is every creature food?

"For Everything created by God is good", but does it make every creature food?

For example if everything is food, could you pray over cocaine and make it food? Whether it is healthy or not?

How about poisonous substances?

Can you eat them?

After all every creature of God is good.

What or who makes food acceptable?

What is food?

Did Jesus make all food clean?

"Because it does not enter his heart but his stomach, and is eliminated, thus purifying all foods?" (Mark 7:19)

Eat The Colors

If, by this statement Jesus made all food clean, then why does God punish people for eating unclean animals in the last days?

"And I saw, coming out of the mouth of the dragon and out of the mouth of the beast and out of the mouth of the false prophet, three unclean spirits like frogs" (Revelation 16:13)

"For behold, the LORD will come with fire and with His chariots, like a whirlwind, to render His anger with fury, and His rebuke with flames of fire. For by fire and by His sword the LORD will judge all flesh; and the slain of the LORD shall be many. 'Those who sanctify themselves and purify themselves, to go to the gardens after an idol in the midst, eating swine's flesh and the abomination and the mouse, shall be consumed together,' says the LORD" (Isaiah:66:15-17)

Kwame Frimpong

Here is my opinion:

These questions are not easy to answer simply because in the New Testament era, God does not tell his children what to eat or not to eat; in the Old Testament He did. Each one is responsible for eating healthy or not.

The New Testament does not abolish the Jewish diet. Neither does it impose it on anyone under the New Covenant. The Jewish diet does not make you any less or any more spiritual. The message is clear that God has given man two major responsibilities as we have stated before:

(1)   God has given you the responsibility to take care of your health

(2)   God has given you the ability to choose, the same way he gave the freedom of choice to Adam and Eve. God wants you to exercise your freedom concerning your health.

Eat The Colors

"For one believes he may eat all things, but he who is weak eats only vegetables. Let not him who eats despise him who does not eat, and let not him who does not eat judge him who eats; for God has received him" (Romans 14:2-3)

Adam and Eve were given permission to eat from any tree, including the tree of life. "And the Lord God commanded the man, saying, "Of every tree of the garden you may freely eat." (Genesis 2:17)
Adam and Eve had the freedom to choose from all kinds of trees. Including the tree of life. They exercised their choice in a bad way. They never ate from the tree of life. God drove them from the Garden and protected the tree. It just stood there. But it had life in it! Had they eaten from that tree they would have lived

forever. They chose to eat junk. The two wrong choices they made were:

a.   They failed to eat from the tree of life

b.   They ate from the tree of death from which they had been forbidden to eat from.

Results: The end result of their disobedience was death. This is the same problem we are facing 6000 years later. We are using our freedom of choice in the wrong direction. The end result is PREMATURE DEATH.

CHAPTER 11:

8 THINGS YOU SHOULD KNOW ABOUT TAKING CARE OF YOU

DO NOT EAT ONLY FOR TASTE, BUT FOR HEALTH

Why do you eat?

Everyone must answer the question, why do we eat? Some people eat just because they feel hungry. Others eat because food tastes good. Still others eat as a coping mechanism when undergoing stress. Whatever your reason is for eating will determine your overall health. If you fail to know the answer to why you eat, you will fall for anything. But if you are able to understand the reasons behind your choices,

Kwame Frimpong

you will be in a better mental position to eat a healthy diet.

1.   Stop being selfish

A lot of people do not know that the reason they can't take good care of their health is due to the fact that they are selfish. I know you probably feel uncomfortable right now, but let me explain. Often people who do not care about their health do not think that family members are concerned about them. They fail to realize that loved ones do not want to see them get sick or die. Your children want to see you in good health for a long time. It is not all about you! God, friends and family matter. You matter to them!

        I was talking to someone who was overweight and his condition never seemed to bother him. It was getting to the point where his medical doctor had become very concerned. Unfortunately, he had not woken up to the reality that his health was at stake. I asked him if he really wanted a change in his life but his answer was something to the effect that "whatever happens will happen." I explained to him that if he cared about his family; parents, siblings and friends, he would realize that people need him here on earth. On the other hand, if all he thinks about is himself alone, then he is being selfish.

2.   Have time for your health

Take time to have time or you may need to have time when you do not have time. To have time you must make time or you may want to have time when there is no time.

There is time for everything under the sun and that includes having time for your health. Not having enough time for your health is not an excuse. God has given time to everyone. While we may not have the same social status as everyone else, all of us have the same 24 hours in a day. The rich, poor, high class, Caucasian, black, middle class, low class and everyone else all have the same amount of time. The most important thing is how you manage your time. This is why David prayed: "So teach us to number our days, That we may gain a heart of wisdom" (Psalm 90:12)

The one common challenge for most people is not seeming to have time to take better care of themselves. Our jobs, friends, families, church programs and all the other "stuff" seem to take all our time. Eating right? Exercising? Juicing? Smoothies? Not possible. All these are legitimate excuses, but the question still remains the same. You need to make the time.

3.   Stop the excuse

Eating healthy is too expensive! Wrong! Pay the price now or pay a much higher price later. If you think taking care of yourself by eating right now is too expensive, then wait and see what happens when you put all that junk in your system! You will soon find out that the price is actually higher for eating junk all the time and ignoring your health.

You cannot succeed in anything without paying a price. The cheaper the price, the less the value. When it comes to health, people often hide themselves in the name of "Oh, it is too expensive!" The truth of the matter is, eating junk is really more expensive.

4. Avoid taking advantage of God

Of all the excuses I see in the body of Christ regarding taking care of your body, the most serious of all in my opinion is taking advantage of God. It is true that our God is a healer. He has promised to heal us through his word, his blood, and his name. There is also power in prayer and God is still in his healing business. However, for us to live any way we choose and expect God to heal us is not walking in wisdom. It is counterproductive and lacks true faith.

5. Treat your system the same way you treat your teeth

If you are like most people, you probably brush your teeth once or twice a day. It does not feel good to eat without first brushing your teeth. Even after a nap you may feel like brushing your teeth. Perhaps we need to answer the question, why do we brush at all? Is it just sort of second nature? You just wake up and automatically brush your teeth? Or is it just so your teeth will look better to people? You know, I am not sure what your reasons are, but I think that for health reasons you need to brush your teeth at least once a day.

Don't you think we need to cleanse our system the same way? Is it because you do not see what is happening in your internal body system that you really do not care? That is, until your doctor says something bad is happening to you? If we had the ability to see what fruit and veggies do inside us I think we would eat fruit to cleanse and veggies to strengthen our system. Have you ever wondered what would happens if your kitchen were left unclean for two months? How could you use your kitchen? Do you know that your body or system needs constant cleansing? Start today!

6.   Your decisions about what you eat make the difference between health and sickness

"And the LORD God commanded the man, saying, "You may surely eat of every tree of the garden, 17 but of the tree of the knowledge of good and evil you shall not eat, for in the day that you eat[a] of it you shall surely die."(Genesis 2:16-17)

From this passage of scripture we know that Adam and Eve ate from the forbidden tree and this was the cause of their downfall. The question is why did they do that? What caused them to desire the food that killed? How come Eve was not closer to the tree of life?

Eat The Colors

Before we criticize them for eating from the forbidden tree we should consider our own lives. Are we not doing the same thing? Are we not eating what I call "dead" foods? Many people are literally losing their lives because of all the junk they are putting in their systems. The temptation is greater today because of the way junk foods are packaged and advertised.

A couple of years ago, Fransisca, a good friend of mine, told me about her co-worker Dorcas, (not her real name), who had just been diagnosed with stomach cancer. Dorcas hated drinking water. To her, water tasted awful. Her drink of choice became sodas, and she really enjoyed soda a lot. One day someone saw her holding a bottle of water and asked her, "What happened to you? You never drink water!" Dorcas replied, "I need to change my diet." Well, several weeks later Fransica was told that

Dorcas had been diagnosed with stomach cancer.

I am sure you know people who would rather spend their money and time on food that does nothing but hurt the body.

7.   Embrace the garden life- Live like a gardener

God put our first parents in a garden. I am not sure why he did not put them in a house or a palace or castle instead, but they lived a long time in the garden. He could have put them in a castle, a house or inside a rock. But why a garden? I think it is an important question. The environment you live in is very important. If it is toxic, it can affect your overall health. God, knowing the duties he gave to man and the responsibility given to him, put him in an environment he could function in very well. In order for you to have a good frame of mind to be able to accomplish anything, you need a healthy environment.

Our whole life is compared to gardening. God our Creator was the first gardener. He planted Adam and Eve in a beautiful Garden called Eden. Jesus also testified to this:

"I am the true vine, and my Father is the gardener" (John 15:1) NIV

In every garden seeds are planted and watered so they will grow and beautify the garden. In the same way, bad seeds can also be planted and grow, sharing the nutrients of the good seeds and this results in killing the good seeds or stopping them from growing. In all our lives, whether we like it or not, good seeds of good food are planted in our bodies and in the same way, bad seeds of bad food are also being planted in our system. The bad seeds keep on destroying the good seeds, thereby affecting our health negatively.

This is why when God told me to plant more good seeds into my system to replace the space that the bad seeds were taking, I got the message. Think about it this way, every time you eat you are sowing a seed in your body garden. Pretty soon you will see the effect because the seed will grow. Have you ever eaten and immediately after that you felt feverish? It could be the fruit of the bad seed of food you just planted in your garden.

Some people do not even pay attention to their body garden. I remember when I was a child I had a garden. Every now and then I would inspect it to see if there were weeds growing because I knew weeds would destroy the good crop. If I found any, I immediately removed them. When I found out that table salt was the cause of my migraines, I stopped eating table salt. Period!

In the same way, God commanded the man to take care of the garden in the Old Testament:

"The Lord God placed the man in the Garden of Eden as its gardener, to tend and care for it." (Genesis 2:15) TLB

He now gives us even a greater command in the New Testament to take care of our health:

"For no one ever hated his own flesh, but nourishes and cherishes it, just as the Lord does the church." (Ephesians 5:29)

God desires our lives on earth to be healthy, as a garden, Isaiah prophesied:

Kwame Frimpong

"For as the earth brings forth its bud, As the garden causes the things that are sown in it to spring forth, So the Lord God will cause righteousness and praise to spring forth before all the nations." (Isaiah 61:11)

What I mean by "embracing the garden life" is that there are so many lessons we could learn from the garden life. Here are few of them.

There are eight things God showed me in the garden that are connected to our health. I believe that if you practice these eight things, your health will improve greatly.

1. Connect with the source. Obeying God's word (God)

"But of the tree of the knowledge of good and evil you shall not eat, for in the day that you eat of it you shall surely die." (Genesis 2:17)

Just like every plant in a garden needs sunlight to grow strong, be healthy and bear fruit, we need the light of God's word to remain spiritually healthy. It is only by staying strong in his word and having an on-going personal relationship with his word, the Bible and with the living word, Jesus, that our lives will be meaningful, rich and productive. You may argue that many people who are not connected to the Source and don't know Jesus are leading fruitful and productive lives. That may be true to some degree. However, without the light of Jesus, and his forgiveness which leads to salvation, the meaning found in this life ends at death's door. For those of us who are saved through the precious blood of Jesus, death holds no fear. We will go on to live eternally in the light of God's love.

2. Eat raw food (fruit and veggies)

"And God said, "See, I have given you every herb that yields seed which is on the face of all the earth, and every tree whose fruit yields seed; to you it shall be for food" (Genesis 1:29)

Fruits and vegetables are excellent sources of vitamins, minerals, complex carbohydrates, fiber, and other food substances, such as phytochemicals. Research suggests that phytochemicals may protect us against heart disease and some types of cancer. Fruits and vegetables give you high nutrition and low calories. They have enormous therapeutic value with their rich nutritional composition, high fiber and water content and boost immunity, improve stamina and protect us from several health problems. Research shows diets containing substantial amounts of varied vegetables and fruits reduce chances of cancer by 20 per cent and of stroke and cardio vascular disease by 60 per cent.- (Bennett, Coleman & Co. Ltd.)

3. Water: There was a lot of water in the Garden for only two people

"Now a river went out of Eden to water the garden, and from there it parted and became four riverheads." (Genesis 2:10)

Water is fundamental part of our lives. It is easy to forget how completely we depend on it. Human survival is dependent on water. Water has been ranked by experts as second only to oxygen as essential for life. The average adult body is 55 to 75 percent water. Two-thirds of your body weight is water (40 to 50 quarts). A human embryo is more than 80 percent water.

Kwame Frimpong

A newborn baby is 74 percent water. Every day your body must replace 2 1/2 quarts of water. The water you drink literally becomes you! Aside from aiding in digestion and absorption of food, water regulates body temperature and blood circulation, carries nutrients and oxygen to cells, and removes toxins and other wastes.

4. Exercising (walking), breathing meditation (cool of the day). Relaxation: The sights, smells, and sounds of the garden are said to promote relaxation and reduce stress

It is frequently stated that the easiest way to remain healthy is to walk. Walking requires no prescription, and there are no risks or side effects.

Here are some benefits of walking:

(1)   Walking boosts the blood circulation

(2)   Weight management.

(3)   Control of blood pressure

(4)   Lowers the risk of a stroke

(5)   Lowers risk of heart attack

(6)   Reduces level of 'bad' cholesterol: Low-density lipoproteins (LDL or bad cholesterol

(7)   Risk of breast cancer is reduced: A 'Nurses Health Study' has shown that regular exercise cuts the risk of breast cancer by a half.

(8)   Control of diabetes type 2.

(9)   Reduced risk of hip and lower limb fracture

(10)   Miscellaneous benefits: The list is endless. Among many other important benefits of regular walking indicated by studies are that walking lowers stress levels, brings back pain relief, improves sleep, reduces depression and elevates overall mood, strengthens muscles and bones, and lengthens life span.

5. HEALTHY RELATIONSHIPS

"And the Lord God said, "It is not good that man should be alone; I will make him a helper comparable to him." (Genesis 2:18)

God, in his awesome power and wisdom, knows that relationships are good for us. Our friends and family, brothers and sisters in the kingdom help our relationship to God to develop. By serving other people, we show our love and gratitude for all God has done for us. By forgiving others, we feel ever more thankful for the depth of God's love in forgiving us. In our need, we provide others with the opportunity to serve their Lord. Healthy relationships make us happier, healthier people.

6. Quality sleep

"And the Lord God caused a deep sleep to fall on Adam, and he slept; and He took one of his

ribs, and closed up the flesh in its place"
(Genesis 2:21)

It's important to give your body time to rest.
Studies have been done that the right amount
of sleep can promote weight loss. In fact, too
little sleep may make it difficult to lose weight.
God never meant for us to spend the better
part of the day in bed, but he did create our
bodies with the need for rest. A lack of sleep
can cause decreased concentration, depression
and increased anxiety. Try to unplug and
disconnect from all your electronic devices at
least an hour or two before you go to bed.
Resist the urge to check "one last time" for a
text message or an email. It can wait until
morning.

All the electronics our brains and our
eyes are exposed to over the course of a day
create an enormous amount of stimulation.

Your brain needs time to unwind! Avoid exercising too close to bedtime also. Exercise cause adrenaline to be released, and this is something you can do without when you're trying to relax. Avoid caffeine after your evening meal. Even small amounts of chocolate can affect some people's sleep.

7. Fresh air and sunshine

And they heard the sound of the Lord God walking in the garden in the cool of the

day

(Genesis 3:8)

God placed Adam and Eve together in the Garden of Eden and he's given us all of creation to enjoy as well. We need fresh air and sunshine to be healthy. The air we breathe inside our homes is much more toxic than much of the air we're exposed to outside. Our carpets and furniture even give off fumes that can make us sick! If you are housebound and can't get outside, open a window just for a few minutes and enjoy the fresh cool breeze. Sit by a warm sunny window and feel the warmth of God's love.

At certain times of the year it can be difficult to spend too much time outside. It's either too hot or too cold. Plan your schedule to take advantage of the cool morning or take a moonlit gentle walk with your spouse or your four-legged companion. Enjoy the beauty of God's creation. It can give you a new perspective on life.

Remember this: the Lord God Almighty, the One Who is and Who is to come, Who slung the stars into space and can count all the grains of sand on a thousand beaches, knows your very name! He is still is control of the universe and is certainly in control of your life.

8. Your God-given assignment

"Then the Lord God took the man and put him in the Garden of Eden to tend and keep it. (Genesis 2:15)

God has given each of us an assignment. Each day of our life brings something to do. Even if we've been retired from our career for 30 years and counting. Even if we haven't started kindergarten yet. Each of us is on a mission from heaven. What gives your life meaning? What gets you out of bed in the morning? Having a purpose bigger than yourself, working towards a goal that is something more precious than the next shinny toy leads to improved health. If you are a banker, be the best banker you can be. If you are a student, be the best student you can be. Maybe you are a father, or an ambassador at the United Nations. Maybe you work at a grocery store. Maybe you live in a nursing home and need help to take a bath. Be whatever it is you are to the glory of God. Remember this: you will make mistakes. Your sins are as red as scarlet. No matter how hard you try, your sinful flesh, the world and satan himself will attempt to knock you down and make you want to give up. You may say that you don't deserve a second chance. Neither did Peter. Or Paul. Or Moses. Or Abraham. I didn't either. But Jesus died, so that we could be forgiven, every single time we make a mistake and ask for a chance to start over. Every day, get out of bed and make it your purpose to use your day for the glory of the One who died to make you his very own child. To God the Father and to Jesus Christ be all the Glory!

Kwame Frimpong

You do not have to have a garden to have the benefit of a gardener. You can practice the 8 things and enjoy:

Stress relief: A recent study in the Netherlands suggests that gardening can fight stress even better than other relaxing leisure activities. "By reintroducing these bacteria in the environment, that may help to alleviate some of these problems," Lowry says.

Exercise: Gardening gets you out in the fresh air and sunshine -- and it also gets your blood moving.

Brain health: Some research suggests that the physical activity associated with gardening can help lower the risk of developing dementia. The sights, smells, and sounds of the garden are said to promote relaxation and reduce stress.

Eat The Colors

Nutrition: Not surprisingly, several studies have shown that gardeners eat more fruits and vegetables than their peers. "People who are growing food tend to eat healthy," says Brown. "The work that we do here with kids demonstrates it on a daily basis, throughout the seasons."

SOME EXAMPLES OF BIBLE FOODS

We remember the fish which we ate freely in Egypt, the cucumbers, the melons, the leeks, the onions, and the garlic (Number 11:5)

Seasonings, Spices and Herbs
- Anise (Matthew 23:23)
- Coriander (Exodus 16:31;
- Numbers 11:7)

Kwame Frimpong

- Cinnamon (Exodus 30:23; Revelation 18:13)
- Cumin (Isaiah 28:25; Matthew 23:23)
- Dill (Matthew 23:23)
- Garlic (Numbers 11:5)
- Mint (Matthew 23:23; Luke 11:42)
- Mustard (Matthew 13:31)
- Rue (Luke 11:42)

Fruits and Nuts

- Apples (Song of Solomon 2:5)
- Almonds (Genesis 43:11; Numbers 17:8)
- Dates (2 Samuel 6:19; 1 Chronicles 16:3)
- Figs (Nehemiah 13:15; Jeremiah 24:1-3)
- Grapes (Leviticus 19:10; Deuteronomy 23:24)
- Melons (Numbers 11:5; Isaiah 1:8)
- Olives (Isaiah 17:6; Micah 6:15)
- Pistachio Nuts (Genesis 43:11)

Eat The Colors

- Pomegranates (Numbers 20:5; Deuteronomy 8:8)
- Raisins (Numbers 6:3; 2 Samuel 6:19)
- Sycamore Fruit (Psalm 78:47; Amos 7:14)

Vegetables and Legumes

- Beans (2 Samuel 17:28; Ezekiel 4:9)
- Cucumbers (Numbers 11:5)
- Gourds (2 Kings 4:39)
- Leeks (Numbers 11:5)
- Lentils (Genesis 25:34; 2 Samuel 17:28; Ezekiel 4:9)
- Onions (Numbers 11:5)

Grains

- Barley (Deuteronomy 8:8; Ezekiel 4:9)
- Bread (Genesis 25:34; 2 Samuel 6:19; 16:1; Mark 8:14)

Kwame Frimpong

- Corn (Matthew 12:1) (refers to "grain" such as wheat or barley)
- Flour (2 Samuel 17:28; 1 Kings 17:12)
- Millet (Ezekiel 4:9)
- Spelt (Ezekiel 4:9)
- Unleavened Bread (Genesis 19:3; Exodus 12:20)
- Wheat (Ezra 6:9; Deuteronomy 8:8)

Fish

- Matthew 15:36
- John 21:11-13

Miscellaneous

- Eggs (Job 6:6; Luke 11:12)
- Grape Juice (Numbers 6:3)
- Honey (Exodus 33:3; Deut 8:8; Judges 14
- Olive Oil (Ezra 6:9; Deuteronomy 8:8)
- Vinegar (Ruth 2:14; John 19:29)

CHAPTER 12:

EASY STEPS FOR WEIGHT LOSS

Losing weight can be very challenging but it should not be. I believe that as you apply these easy steps, you can see immediate changes.

W E I G H T

(1)   W- walking 2-3 miles daily can make a significant difference in your life.

(2)   W- water drink a minimum of 64 ounce of water daily or divide your body weight

by 2 and drink water equal to half your body weight

(3)   E- eat a lot of fruits and veggies

(4)   I- involve someone who is also on the weight loss program to inspire you

(5)   G- get rid of sugars, fried foods, junk

(6)   H -have fun! Try new and different veggies recipes

(7)   T- trainer, if you can afford one, get a trainer

WALKING

I cannot over-emphasize the importance of walking if you are serious about losing weight. Losing weight does not have to mean investing a lot of money in expensive equipment. You do not have to join a gym or buy special clothes. All it requires is a desire to get to a better place than where you are now.

Maybe two miles a day sounds like an insurmountable goal. If it does, aim for a distance you can reach. Or set aside a specific length of time per day you will walk. When you reach that goal, challenge yourself by setting a new one. It doesn't matter where you start, but you have to start somewhere. You can take a walk on your lunch break at work. You can walk before you get ready for work in the morning. You can walk after dinner in the evening. Remember, this isn't vigorous exercise that might make it difficult for you to fall asleep. This type of walking is not meant to make your heart race or make it hard for you to breathe.

Listen to music or just enjoy the scenery around you. Many local libraries have audio books you can listen to while you walk. You could "read" many books this way, listen to sermons or read through the Bible this way. Listen for what God is saying to you. Spend the time praying or meditating on your day.

As you get in the habit of walking, it will get easier. First, because as you start to lose pounds, there will be less weight for your body to carry, but also because you will build strength and endurance. Your muscles will grow stronger: leg muscles, back, abdominal and chest muscles, but also your heart, which is also a muscle.

Walking not only burns calories to help you lose weight, it also burns off stress. Life is full of pressure that causes anxiety and tension and trying to lose weight makes it even more stressful. Walking helps by causing the body to release "feel good" hormones. It helps you calm down and deal with problems more effectively.

WATER

Water is the second "W" in "WEIGHT" for weight loss. I have already explained many times how important water is to your health in general. It is also vital to weight loss. Burning fat is the liver's job. When you aren't drinking enough water, the liver has to help the kidneys with their work. This makes the liver less efficient at its job of fat of burning extra fat.

Water is also vital in the process of digesting your food and absorbing all the nutrients found in your diet. When you're dieting, you need all the nutrition from the food you're eating. Water also helps prevent constipation and it helps to flush away the toxic waste that is created when the liver burns excess fat. It's nature's own original detox.

Kwame Frimpong

Water can also suppress your appetite. It will make you feel full and you're less like to over-eat if you make sure to drink plenty of water throughout the day. Many times people will mistake hunger for thirst. If you're having trouble drinking enough water here are some ideas you can try:

• Before you eat or drink anything else, coffee included, start your morning with a glass of water.

• Before every meal, before you take your first bite, drink a glass of water

• Before you take your daily walk, and again when you're finished, drink a glass of water. Take a bottle of water along on your walk and sip on it while you walk, especially as you increase the distance and time you spend walking. It's especially important to stay well-hydrated during physical activity

• Any time you are watching television, keep a bottle or glass of water beside you. Every time your program takes a commercial break, take a drink.

EAT A LOT OF FRUITS AND VEGGIES

I have talked at length in this book about the importance of eating fruits and veggies. They are vital to healthy living. You need to eat the colors! Try to eliminate all processed foods from your diet. This means anything that contains sugar or artificial sweeteners. Substitute the natural sweetness and flavors found in foods and spices. Keep a variety of fresh fruit on hand so when the urge to snack strikes, you have something convenient to satisfy your hunger and don't reach for just anything. If you just have choice available, you might get bored and be more easily drawn off course.

Besides the usual carrots and celery sticks, keep a wide variety of healthy snacks visible and ready to eat. Cucumber slices, fresh broccoli, fresh cauliflower, radishes, orange slices, apples, bananas, fresh tomatoes, peaches, berries, melon cubes, pineapple chunks, tangerines, grapes, cherries, avocado slices. Keep lettuce and greens available for so you can toss together a quick salad anytime you get hungry. Try putting your fruits on your salads as well as your veggies. Frozen peas add variety to salad, or try snow peas.

You can make frozen smoothies that are cool and refreshing using frozen fruits and veggies. They are so delicious and so healthy. They are tons of nutritious goodness in a single serving; Fiber, mineral, vitamins and lots of healthy natural juice without any added sugar or artificial flavorings, preservatives or chemicals.

Involve someone who is on the weight loss program with you

Anything you do with someone else always seems like less work and more fun. If you have a person who you can be accountable to and who is accountable to you, your chance of success increases. Avoid comparing yourself with each other and set your own goals because God has created each of us to be unique, but support and provide encouragement to each other. Don't forget to pray for one another.

Maybe you could find a time to walk together or compare notes on recipes you've found. You may even be able to share shopping trips to a special market you've found. It may be more economical to buy fresh produce in larger quantities and share between the two of you.

GET RID OF SUGAR, FRIED FOODS AND JUNK

Fruits and vegetables should make up about half of the total amount of food you heat. The other food you eat should be divided equally between proteins and whole grain foods. This leaves very little room for a small amount of fat and no room for fried foods, sugar, sweets or junk. Your body doesn't need these.

Choose lean proteins like poultry without the skin, fish, beans and fat-free dairy products. Try to limit your intake of dairy to 2-3 servings per day. Don't forget that processed meats like ham, bacon and summer sausage are generally loaded with salt and many of these foods are far from lean. Limit servings of red meat to one per week. Beans are a great source of protein. Nuts also contain protein.

Whole grains are grains that have not been refined so you get the entire seed, including the bran and the germ. None of the vital nutrition has been lost in the process of crushing, grinding or cooking the grain. Choose whole grain cereals, whole grain breads and avoid white flour and white rice. These foods fill you up faster and keep you from getting hungry because it takes your body longer to digest them.

HAVE FUN!

This is important! Eating fruit and veggies doesn't have to be boring. When you do your weekly shopping, try choosing one new food and find a recipe to try using it. You don't have to buy a large quantity or try anything extravagant. Ask the butcher or the produce manager for hints or tips on how to prepare food you are unfamiliar with or search online for new recipes.

TRAINER

This is the last letter in the WEIGHT approach for weight loss. If you can afford one, a trainer can help you customize a program for weight loss and a diet approach that fits your individual body type, health and fitness profile and your lifestyle. Your trainer will work with you to set goals that are realistic and then help you monitor your progress and provide encouragement and support.

CHAPTER 13: CONCLUSION

I hope Eat the Colors has been a blessing to you. It is my prayer that God will use the information I have provided about the blessings he has granted to me to bless you with success on your path toward better health. May you feel his love more deeply and grow ever closer to Him as your Lord and Savior. May He endow you with the grace to take care of your temple which is your body.

Now to Him who is able to do exceedingly abundantly above all that we ask or think, according to the power that works in us, to Him be glory in the church by Christ Jesus to all generations, forever and ever. Amen. (Ephesians 3:20)

My Healthy Habits

Kwame Frimpong

(1)   Restless Leg Syndrome

         Wear Socks Compression to bed
         Drink Chamomile tea
         Drink Apple Cidar Vinegar

(2)   Migraines
         I   avoid   eating   the   following
completely.

              Table salt
              Sodas
              Caffeine
              Sausage

         Find out what triggers your migraines:

Eat The Colors

What did you eat prior to experiencing the migraines?

What did you do prior to experiencing the migraines?

Your answers to these questions could give you a clue about what triggers your migraines

(3)   Chronic idiopathic thrombocytopenia and leukopenia

              Juice twice weekly with a lot of spinach

              Eat a lot of Veggies

              Drink a lot of water

(4)   Insomnia

       Walk 3 to 4 miles daily and 6 miles every now and then

My typical day

Kwame Frimpong

I drink 16 ounce of water with lemon daily
Follow by green tea with 8 ounce of water and
honey
I eat a lot of almond seed daily
A lot of veggies daily

(5)   Blood pressure

Drink half lemon and 16 ounce of water daily

My Favorite Smoothie
½ apple/Cucumber

½ banana/full cup pineapple/Mangoes

Kale/Spinach

Eat The Colors

About 2 or 3 Carrot

Strawberry or any of the berries

Broccoli
My favorite Juicing
Carrot

Spinach

Mangoes/pineapple

Asparagus

Beet roots

Apple/Kiwi

Kwame Frimpong

Questions and answers

1.   Should I stop taking my medications because I am eating healthy?

Ans: No

2.   I am so addicted to junk food, how can I stop?

Ans: You can prepare healthy food that looks and taste like junk i.e. baked carrot fries and baked sweet potatoes fries

3.   How can I stick to a healthy lifestyle?

Ans: Get a buddy who is also on the program

Que:

Eat The Colors

God changed Noah's diet after the flood and permitted to eat meat,

"Everything that lives and moves about will be food for you. Just as I gave you the green plants, I now give you everything".

I love beef are you saying we should not eat beef?

Ans:

The original plan by God for man was to be vegetarian (Gen 1:29). But after the flood when all the vegetation was destroyed, God permitted man to eat meat and then again under the law He commands them concerning clean and unclean meat (Lev 11)

Here is my opinion

In the beginning when God created man to live forever, His original plan for man was to be vegetarian (Gen 1:29)

Kwame Frimpong

After the flood when man's condition had changed because of sin, God allowed man to eat everything he so desires (Gen 9:3)

Now when God decided to use Israel as a model to bless all the families of the earth, he gave them instructions concerning food (Lev 11)

In conclusion

We are free to eat meat (Gen 9:3) therefore enjoy your meat, however you must know what meat is good for your health and the healthy way to prepare it.

Watch this: On several occasions God mentions fruit, vegetables or leafs for food (Gen 1:29, Gen 9:3, Ezekiel 47:12 and Revelation 22:2) but when it comes to meat God becomes highly selective

Eat The Colors

In his book "what you don't know may be killing you" and "walking in divine health" Dr. Don Colbert offers good advice on meat in take, he tells you what meat is good for you and what is not.

I have started and stopped several times, how can I maintain consistency?
Ans: Get a buddy who is on the program and get inspired by reading books about health

Watchword: Moderation,

Kwame Frimpong

Pastor Kwame Frimpong is the founder of Breakthrough in Christ Ministry, a multimedia ministry with the purpose of reaching the world for Jesus. He is an Author, ordained minister, national speaker and songwriter, Humility, compassion and integrity best describe the ministry of Pastor Kwame, with a high energy, down-to-earth approach while uniquely blending practical wisdom with God's Word, Kwame's messages couples with a heart of compassion for the broken and downtrodden has led many to pursue a personal relationship with God.

Pastor Kwame attended Action Faith Bible College in Accra-Ghana, whose chancellor is Bishop Nicholas Duncan-

Williams. He is an ordained minister and currently, he is continuing his studies at Liberty University. Pastor Kwame is an insightful Bible teacher, songwriter and passionate motivational speaker. His heartfelt desire is to see believers recognize and defeat the enemy in their personal lives and in their churches.

Since 1989, Pastor Kwame has been in full time ministry teaching extensively in Africa, Europe and the United States. Hundreds of individuals and families have benefited from both his Pastoral and Family counseling work. Kwame Frimpong TV Ministry "Breakthrough Today" has been seen in 200 countries and 100 million homes in the US through the "The Word TV Network"

Pastor Kwame has appeared on the following national TV Stations; CTN Television Florida,

Kwame Frimpong

SBN Television New Mexico, TCT Television Buffalo NY, Its Time for Hope (Freda Crews) Spartanburg SC

Kwame is originally from Ghana, West Africa, though he has been residing in the U.S.A. for the past 18 years. He currently resides in Charlotte, NC with his spouse, Mary and their three daughters Esther, Gloria, and Edna. He is available to speak at churches, seminars and youth retreats. His upbeat motivational messages include four books, The healing of the heart "Overcoming Offenses", "It's Not Your Fault", "Breaking Through to the Real You, 15 Laws of Breakthrough" and "Eat the colors Stop the killers" which has blessed many and continues to be a blessing.

He can be reached by e-mail at info@breakthroughtoday.org or

Eat The Colors

kwamebook@yahoo.com or you can visit him
online@ www.breakthroughtoday.org

www.ingramcontent.com/pod-product-compliance
Lightning Source LLC
Chambersburg PA
CBHW050128280326
41933CB00010B/1293